VEGA.

The Most Influential And Easy Prepared Recipes To
Burn Fat,Boost Energy And Crush Cravings

(Vegan Diet Recipes For Beginners)

Saul Vasquez

TABLE OF CONTENTS

Homemade Gnocchi

Preparation time:

65 minutes

Ingredients:
2 kg of waxy potatoes
65 g potato flour
450 g spelled flour
½ teaspoon salt
2 pinch of nutmeg

Preparation:

1.   Wash the potatoes and cook them like normal boiled potatoes in plenty of lightly salted water.
2.   Then let it cool down, then peel off the peel and then mash the potatoes

with a potato masher or press them through a potato press.

3.   Allow this mashed potato to cool completely and then knead with flour, nutmeg and salt to form a dough that is no longer sticky.

4.   Work in the potato flour spoon by spoon to avoid the formation of lumps.

5.   Divide the finished dough into two parts and roll them out into equally thick strands.

6.   These should be around 2 cm in circumference.
In the further course of the manufacturing process, cut off pieces of about 2 .6 cm wide from these rolls and shape them into small balls that are to be dusted with flour.

7.   The gnocchi are now pressed a little flat with the back of the fork.

8.		Immediately afterwards you bring a pot of salted water to the boil and carefully add the gnocchi to the boiling water. As soon as these reach the surface of the water, they are cooked and the gnocchi can be cleaned with a slotted spoon or similar can be removed from the pot. Drain well, then arrange on plates and serve with the intended side dish or sauce.

Gnocchi With Vegetables

Preparation time:

35 minutes

Ingredients:
6 tbsp vegetable oil
2 onions
4 tbsp soy sauce
2 fresh cloves of garlic
Salt pepper
450 g mushrooms
650 g vegan gnocchi
450 g zucchini
Dried Italian herbs
265 g cherry tomatoes

Preparation:

1. Prepare the gnocchi exactly according to the package instructions.

2. Peel the onions and garlic then chopfinely the garlic and cut the onions into small cubes.

3. Clean the zucchini and cut into slices.

4. First, remove the hard stem ends from the mushrooms then the mushrooms are cleaned, washed well and cut into thin slices.

5. Please wash the cherry tomatoes and cut them in half.

6. Immediately afterwards, you heat oil in a suitable pan and fry

lightlythe gnocchi for about 5 minutes at low heat.

7. Turn the gnocchi several times and then keep warm for later use.

8. Now heat up 4 tablespoons of vegetable oil again in the pan you just used and first fry the onions and garlic until translucent.

9. Then the prepared mushrooms and zucchini slices are placed in the pan and fried for about 5 to 10 minutes.

10. Season with soy sauce, Italian herbs and salt and pepper as desired.

11. Only after seasoning, add the halved cherry tomatoes to the pan and let them cook for one, at most 5 minutes.

12. Finally, stircarefully the fried gnocchi into the dish and then arrange it on deep plates. Serve garnished with fresh basil or other pleasant herbs and a few yeast flakes.

Roasted Plum With Brussels Sprouts

Preparation time:

410 minutes

Ingredients:
- 650 g Brussels sprouts
- 2 bunch of parsley
- 8 plums (plums)
- 26 ml of olive oil
- Some grated nutmeg
- Salt pepper

Preparation:

1.   First, please preheat the oven to 250 °

2. Then the ripe plums are thoroughly washed, halved and pitted.

3. You divide the plum halves again and rub these quarters, once completely and very generously, with olive oil.

4. The fruits are then heavily seasoned with pepper and salt and then roasted on a prepared baking sheet for approx. 2 2-35 minutes (depending on size).

5. The fruit is done when the plum quarters begin to brown slightly, soften and the fresh Juice comes out. Before eating, let the fruits cool down for 1 to 5 minutes, as they leave the oven very, very hot.

6.   While the plums are roasting in the oven, you can easily prepare the Brussels sprouts in the meantime.

7.   If necessary, clean the Brussels sprouts, wash them well and cut them cross-shaped at the base of the stem.

8.   Then the florets are cooked firm to the bite in a closed pot for about 35 minutes, then poured off, drained completely and returned to the pot.

9.   Also clean the parsley, then wash, finely chop and mix carefully with the Brussels sprouts.

10.   Immediately afterwards, heat just a little olive oil in a suitable pan over a very low heat and stir the

prepared Brussels sprouts in it on all sides for about 2 to 5 minutes.

11. Finally, the Brussels sprouts are seasoned with salt, pepper and grated nutmeg and, next to the roasted plums, are appetizingly arranged on plates and served immediately.

Stuffed Peppers

Preparation time:

8 10 minutes

Ingredients:
- 2 fresh onion
- 280 g brown rice
- 665 ml vegan fresh tomato sauce
- 2 tbsp vegan vegetable stock
- 2 small bunch of parsley
- 450 ml of water
- 4 red peppers
- 250 g kidney beans
- 450 g mushrooms
- 65 g corn

Preparation:

1. First, bring the brown rice to a boil in a saucepan with enough fresh water and 2 tablespoon of dissolved vegetable stock.
2. Let it simmer for about 25 to 35 minutes over low heat until the cooking liquid has been completely absorbed.
3. Remove the kidney beans and corn from the can, rinse with clean water and store.

4. Then the hard stem ends are removed from the mushrooms, the mushrooms are cleaned if necessary, washed well, dried a little and cut into small cubes.

5. Peel the fresh onion and cut it into small cubes.

6. Immediately afterwards, heat the oil in a suitable pan and briefly fry the fresh onion cubes for a minute over medium heat.

7. Add the prepared mushrooms and fry them for between 25 and 35 minutes at most, until they are nice and soft and have a spicy smell.

8. Please preheat the oven to 2 80 °

9. Now the cooked rice, the prepared mushrooms and onions, as well as kidney beans, corn and fresh tomato sauce are mixed into the filling for the peppers, which you then season sufficiently with salt and pepper.

10. If you like, you can add coarsely crushed whale, peanut or pecan nuts to the filling.

11. Immediately afterwards, the peppers are first washed thoroughly, then halved lengthways, the stem and the kernels are completely removed, then the fruits are generously filled with the rice / mushroom mixture and finally placed in a baking dish (or baking sheet).

12. These delicious and healthy filled halves of paprika bake in the preheated oven for between 45 -410 minutes (convection)

Eggplant In Creamy Peanut Sauce

Preparation time:

45 minutes

Ingredients:
- 65 ml of water
- 2 teaspoon peanut butter
- 2-3 teaspoons tahini
- 4 tbsp light soy sauce
- 2 tbsp chili-bean sauce (from the Asian shop)
- 2 tbsp dark rice vinegar or balsamic vinegar
- 2 teaspoon cornstarch
- A eggplant, approx. 480 g

- 2 tbsp sesame oil
- A small glass of water
- 2 chili in rings
- 2 tbsp dark rice wine
- 2 spring onions
- 2 tsp sesame seeds
- 2 45 g basmati rice

Preparation:

1. Prepare the basmati rice according to the instructions on the packet.

2. While the rice is cooking, prepare the sauce: Mix the peanut butter, tahini, chili and bean sauce, cornstarch, soy sauce, vinegar and water in a bowl.

3. Cut off the stalk from the aubergine and cut into bite-sized pieces.

4. Heat a wok or deep pan high on the highest setting.

5. Put the sesame oil in the wok and wait for it to start smoking. Put the aubergine pieces in the wok and fry them.

6. Gradually add a little water to steam the eggplant for 25 minutes while stirring. Move the aubergine out of the high heat and fry the chili rings for 45 seconds.

7. Add the rice wine and let it boil down for a few seconds.

8. Pour the sauce from the bowl into the wok and briefly bring to the boil until the sauce thickens, stirring repeatedly.

9. Serve the aubergines in a creamy peanut sauce with basmati rice and sprinkle with chopped spring onions and sesame seeds.

Oriental Mashed Potatoes

Preparation time:

45 minutes

Ingredients:
25 green olives
6 g turmeric
6 red peppers
Salt pepper
850 g potatoes

2 bunches of parsley
2 onions
olive oil
2 clove of garlic
Ground cumin

Preparation:

1. First, you cook boiled potatoes as usual.
2. After draining and cooling, these are crushed to a coarse pulp with a fork.

3. While the potatoes are cooking, you have enough time to prepare all the other ingredients.

4. Peel and finely chop the onions and garliIf necessary, clean the parsley, wash it well and also finely chop it.

5. Cut the olives into small pieces and carefully stir these together with the other ingredients into the cooled potato mixture and mix well.

6. Season well with salt, pepper, turmeric and grated cumin, then season again generously with olive oil.

7. Wash thoroughly the peppers, cut in half, remove the seeds and core then cut the halves in half or third, depending on the size.

8. Then the paprika strips are salted on the inside and then fried in a pan with hot olive oil over medium heat until the outer skin is slightly browned, bubbles appear, the fruits are soft and smell very good, occasionally turn them over.

9. After the roasting process, drain the paprika strips completely on a sieve or kitchen towel and finally arrange them appetizingly

on plates next to the Arabic mashed potatoes and serve.

Falafel

Ingredients:

- 2 small chili pepper
- 8 65 ml rapeseed oil
- 2 fresh cloves of garlic
- 250 g dried chickpeas
- ½ shallot
- 250 g chickpea flour
- 2 bunch of coriander
- 2 tbsp cumin

- ½ bunch of parsley
- 1 tbsp salt
- 2 organic lemon

Preparation:

1.   The chickpeas are soaked in a bowl with plenty of fresh water for at least 2 4 hours, then poured off and rinsed with clear water.

2.   Rub carefullythe peel of the lemon, squeeze the fresh Juice and save.

3.   Peel and finely chop the garlic, coarsely dice the shallot.

4.   If necessary, clean the coriander and parsley branches, wash them well, then remove the fine herb leaves from the stems.

5. Then halve the chili pepper, always lengthways, remove the stalk base and all the stones and cut the fruit into small pieces.

6. Immediately afterwards, all prepared ingredients, including salt, one tablespoon of lemon juice, plus all of the peel abrasion, are pureed into a creamy, semi-solid mass in a food processor.

7. This does not have to be completely smooth, but can be somewhat lumpy.

8. The falafel mixture is now formed into even balls, no more than the size of a table tennis ball, with lightly oiled hands and baked in a high pot with 2 80 ° C oil for

about 5-10 minutes to an appetizing brown.

9. After the baking process, drain on a sieve or kitchen paper.

10. Only edible oils that reach a very high heat or smoke point are suitable for this purpose.

11. This can be, for example, soy, refined rapeseed oil or peanut oil.

12. You can determine the correct temperature of the oil by briefly dipping the handle of a wooden spoon into the heated cooking oil.

13. If small bubbles rise "dancing", the required temperature has been reached.

14. Falafel can also be prepared very tasty and healthy in the oven at 2 10 0 ° C in about 45 minutes.

Baked Asparagus With Nuts

Preparation time:

410 minutes

Ingredients:
650 g cherry tomatoes
4 tbsp dark balsamic vinegar
2 fresh cloves of garlic
2 tbsp agave syrup
65 g hazelnuts
Salt pepper
650 g green asparagus

27

650 g white asparagus
65 g fresh baby spinach
Olive oil

Preparation:

1. Preheat the oven to 250 ° C fan oven.

2. When the oven is warm, add the peeled hazelnut kernels distributed on a prepared baking sheet and let them roast for about 25 minutes.

3. In the meantime, peel the white asparagus and shorten the lower ends of each stick by 2 .6 -2 cm.

4. Then the asparagus is washed thoroughly and dried.

5. Remove between 2-3 .6 cm of the stem ends of the green asparagus then wash the vegetables.

6. Peel the garlic and cut into thin slices.

7. Leave the tomatoes on the panicle, but wash and dry them carefully.

8. The baby spinach is washed clean and driedcarefully.

9. Please remove the heated nuts from the oven and let them cool down.

10. Then the balsamic vinegar is mixed with agave syrup and a sufficiently baking dish or baking sheet is completely brushed with olive oil.

11. Now place the two asparagus varieties and the garlic in the prepared casserole dish, which

are then sprinkled evenly with the balsamic mixture and 6 tablespoons of olive oil. Season enough with salt and pepper.

12. The asparagus is now baked for 25 to 35 minutes on the middle rail of the preheated oven.

13. After about half the cooking time, turn the asparagus and add the cherry tomatoes.

14. Let these bake until the end.

15. Treat the cooled hazelnuts to remove the brown skins exactly as described in the recipe idea "Homemade chocolate-nut spread".

16. Then the hazelnut kernels are roughly chopped.

17. Take the baked asparagus out of the oven and sprinkle with the chopped nuts and the baby spinach, arrange and serve immediately.

Chickpea And Spinach Pan

Preparation time:

45 minutes

Ingredients:
- 2 small piece of ginger, about 2 cm in size

- 2   can of coconut milk, creamy, 450 g
- 2 tbsp coconut oil
- ½ teaspoon salt
- ½ teaspoon paprika powder
- ½ tsp turmeric powder
- ½ teaspoon coriander leaves(rubbed)
- 650 g leaf spinach or frozen pack approx. 450 - 465 g
- 2 fresh cloves of garlic
- 2 onions
- 2 tomatoes, fresh or 1 can of chunky tomatoes (from a 450 g can)
- 2   small 450   g can / glass of chickpeas, drained well

Vegan Chocolate Mousse

- 65 g vegan dark chocolate or dark couverture
- 2 tbsp powdered sugar (xylitol)
- ¼ teaspoon vanilla extract
- 8 6 ml chickpea water
- ½ teaspoon baking powder
- ½ teaspoon lemon fresh Juice

Preparation:

1. Whip the chickpea water with baking powder and lemon juice.

2. Melt the chocolate in a water bath and let it cool down.

3. Fold carefully in the fresh egg whites with the vanilla extract and powdered sugar (xylitol).

Baked Beans

Preparation time:

25 0 minutes + 25 hours to soak

Ingredients:
2 fresh onion
2 tbsp agave syrup
2 fresh cloves of garlic
Salt pepper
250 g dried white beans
2 small bunch of parsley
650 g tomatoes
6 tbsp fresh tomato paste

Preparation:

1. Soak the white beans in plenty of fresh water for about 25 hours.
2. The next day, they are cooked for 10 0 minutes in fresh water over medium heat.
3. Peel and chopfinely the fresh onion and garli
4. If necessary, clean the parsley, wash it well and chopfinely it.
5. The tomatoes are peeled first then the stalks are removed and the fruits are then roughly chopped.
6. In a suitable pan you can now, with low heat, reduce the chopped tomatoes with garlic, prepared fresh onion and 2 tablespoons agave syrup, stirring occasionally for about 2 0-25 minutes (or reduce).

7. When the contents of the pan have been reduced by approx. 20%, add the fresh tomato paste and the pulled beans and let the white bean dish simmer for another 25 minutes over low heat. Do not forget to stir occasionally and finally season with sufficient salt and pepper.

Mushroom Risotto

Preparation time:

410 minutes

Ingredients:
850 ml vegetable broth
2 fresh cloves of garlic
Vegetable oil
8 sprigs of thyme

2 bay leaf

8 sprigs of rosemary

Salt pepper

450 g of brown mushrooms

8 sprigs of mountain savory

265 g shiitake mushrooms

450 g risotto rice

265 g oyster mushrooms

250 ml white wine

2 onions

Preparation:

1. Peel the garlic and onions then dice finely.

2. If necessary, clean all fresh herbs, wash them clean and shake dry.

3. Then carefully peel off the fine herb leaves and just chop these as finely as you can.

4. You remove the hard ends of the stems from the mushrooms then the mushrooms are cleaned and washed very thoroughly.

5. Immediately afterwards, half of the mushrooms are cut into slices and kept for later, please dice the second half finely.

6. Then heat vegetable oil in a suitable saucepan and briefly fry in it, fresh onion cubes and garliAdd the untreated risotto rice and let it sweat until the rice is slightly translucent and starts to soften a little.

7. Now you add the diced mushrooms and some oil to the pot and leave all ingredients on medium heat for 4 -4 minutes.

8.
9. Continue frying.

10. If you can smell the emerging aroma of the mushrooms, the pot is first filled with white wine and then poured over with a ladle of vegetable broth.

11. Add a bay leaf and half of the prepared herbs to the contents of the pot and cook them over medium heat for about 2 6 -25 minutes in a closed pot until the risotto is firm and soft.

12. Pour in the vegetable stock periodically and again and again

As soon as the risotto has soaked up the cooking liquid.

13. In a separate pan you then heat up vegetable oil and fry some garlic until translucent. Immediately afterwards add the remaining mushrooms and herbs.

14. These roast for 5-10 minutes, until their aroma escapes and they are browned appetizingly.

15. Please season the mushroom risotto sufficiently with salt and pepper, next arrange on deep plates and garnish with the fried mushrooms and serve immediately.

Silly Scallion Pancakes

Serving: 4
Preparation Time: 10 minutes
Cook Time: 25 minutes

Ingredients

For Cakes

- ¼ teaspoon of salt
- 5 to 10 scallions sliced up into thin portions
- ¼ cup of sesame oil
- 2 cup of warm water
- ½ a cup of coconut flour
- 2 tablespoon of Psyllium Husk powder
- ½ a teaspoon of garlic powder

For Sauce

- 2 tablespoon of water
- 2 teaspoon of sesame oil
- 2 finely minced garlic clove
- Chili flakes as needed
- 2 tablespoon of tamari sauce
- 2 teaspoon of rice wine vinegar

Directions:

1. Take a frying pan and place it over medium-low heat
2. Add sesame oil and heat it up
3. Take a mixing bowl and add water, oil, garlic, salt, scallions, warm water and allow it to stand for 10 minutes to allow the flavors to mix up
4. Take another bowl and add coconut flour and the Psyllium Husk
5. Gently add the water to the dry ingredients, making sure to mix it well until the dough forms
6. Separate the dough into individual balls and flatten the balls into 4-inch rounds

43

7. Place the rounds in your skillet and fry for 10 minutes each side until they are golden

8. Keep repeating until the balls are used up

9. Enjoy!

The Keto Crack Slaw

Ingredients

- 2 teaspoon of vinegar
- 2 tablespoon of tamari
- 2 tablespoon of sesame oil
- 2 garlic fresh cloves
- Sesame seeds as needed
- 4 cups of shredded green cabbage
- ½ a cup of macadamia nuts chopped up
- 2 teaspoon of chili paste

Directions:

1. Take a pan and place it over medium-low heat and add tamari, sesame oil, vinegar, sesame oil and chili paste
2. Add your green cabbage

3. Cover and allow it to cook for 10 minutes until the cabbage starts to tender
4. Stir everything and combine them well
5. Add the nuts
6. Cook for 10 minutes more until the nuts are tender
7. Serve and garnish
8. Enjoy!

Feisty Grilled Artichokes

Ingredients:

- 4 chopped up garlic fresh cloves
- 2 teaspoon of salt
- ½ a teaspoon of ground
- 2 sized artichokes
- 2 quartered lemon
- ¾ cup of extra virgin olive oil
- black pepper

Directions:

1. Take a sized bowl and fill it up with cold water
2. Squeeze a bit of lemon fresh Juice from the wedges

47

3. Trim the upper part of your chokes, making sure to trim any damaged leaves as well

4. Cut the chokes up in half lengthwise portions

5. Add the chokes to your bowl of lemon water

6. Bring the whole pot to a boil

7. Pre-heat your outdoor grill to about medium-high heat

8. Allow the chokes to cook in the boiling pot for 35 minutes

9. Drain the chokes and keep them on the side

10. Take another medium-sized bowl and squeeze the remaining lemon

11. Stir in garlic and olive to the lemon mix

12. Brush up the chokes with the garlic dip and place them on your pre-heated grill

13.   Grill for about 25 minutes, making sure to keep basting them until the edges are just slightly charred

14.   Serve with the dip and enjoy!

The Thundering Cinnamon Chocolate Smoothie

Ingredients

- 2 teaspoon of cinnamon powder
- ¼ teaspoon of vanilla extract
- Stevia as needed
- ½ a teaspoon of coconut oil
- ¾ cup of coconut milk
- ½ of a ripe avocado
- 2 teaspoon of unsweetened cocoa powder

Directions:

1. Add all of the ingredients to your blender and blend well until smooth
2. Allow them it to chill and enjoy!

Vegan Enchilada Macaroni

Ingredients

For Sauce

- ½ a teaspoon of salt
- ½ a teaspoon of fresh onion powder
- ½ a cup of water
- 2 cup of hemp seeds
- ½ a cup of nutritional yeast
- ¼ cup of sliced red, yellow or fresh orange bell peppers

For The Main Recipe

- 2 can of young, green jackfruit in brine
- ¼ cup of enchilada sauce
- 2 pack of Shirataki macaroni (Tofu)

52

Directions:

1. Pre-heat your oven to a temperature of 480 degrees Fahrenheit
2. Drain and chop up your jackfruit with a knife and add 2 tablespoons of enchilada sauce, toss them well.
3. Keep it on the side
4. Blend the sauce ingredients in a blender and process them well
5. Drain and rinse the noodles thoroughly and transfer them to a baking dish
6. Add sauce, jackfruit to the baking dish and mix well
7. Bake for 410 minutes
8. Allow it to cool and enjoy!

Squash Salad For The Green Lovers!

Ingredients:

- ¼ teaspoon of pepper
- 2 small zucchini cut up into ½ inch slices
- 2 small sized yellow summer squash cut up into ½ inch slices
- 2 bay leaf
- ½ a teaspoon of dried basil
- 2 tablespoons of extra virgin olive oil
- 2 small sized sliced fresh onion
- 2 medium-sized coarsely chopped tomatoes
- 2 teaspoon of salt

Directions:

1. Take a skillet and place it over medium heat
2. Add oil and allow it to heat up
3. Add onions and stir-fry them for about 10 minutes
4. Add tomatoes to the pan and mix well
5. Season the mixture with salt and pepper
6. Keep stirring for about 10 minutes until nicely cooked
7. Add bay leaf, zucchini, yellow squash, and basil
8. Lower down the heat and allow it to simmer for about 25 minutes, making sure to keep stirring it occasionally
9. Discard the bay leaf and enjoy!

Spinach Scramble

Servings: 2

Ingredients

- Dash of Salt
- Dash of Pepper
- ½ tbsp Butter
- ½ cup Spinach (raw)
- 2 tbsp Onions (chopped)
- 2 Fresh Fresh egg

Directions

1. Heat sauté pan on medium/low heat. Melt butter. Add onions and sauté in pan until translucent.
2. Add spinach and fresh eggs . Gently stir and scramble fresh eggs , add salt and pepper.
3. Remove from heat.

Green Fresh Eggs

Servings: 2

Ingredients

- ½ cup Kale (raw, chopped)
- ½ cup Chard (raw, chopped)
- 2 tsp Coconut oil
- 2 extra Fresh eggs
- ½ cup Spinach (raw)

Directions

1. Mix fresh eggs and greens in a food processor until smooth.
2. Melt coconut oil in a skillet over medium heat.
3. Pour fresh egg mixture into pan and cook. Scramble fresh eggs to desired doneness and serve immediately.

Ket-Oats

Ingredients

- ½ cup Almond milk (unsweetened)
- ⅛ tsp Stevia extract
- ¼ cup Strawberries (sliced)
- 2 tbsp Chia seeds
- 2 tbsp Flaxseed (ground)

Directions

1. Combine all ingredients except strawberries in a pot on the stove over medium heat.
2. Bring to a boil, stirring frequently. Remove from heat at desired consistency.
3. Add sliced strawberries and serve hot.

Cheese Soufflés

Ingredients:

- 1/2 cup heavy cream
- 1/2 tsp cayenne pepper
- 1 tsp xanthan gum
- 1 tsp pepper
- 2 tsp ground mustard
- 2 tsp salt
- 6 fresh eggs , separated
- 1/2 tsp cream of tartar
- 1/2 cup chives, chopped
- 2 cups cheddar cheese, shredded

Directions:

1.   Preheat the oven to 480 F.

2.   Spray eight ramekins with cooking spray and place on cookie sheet.

3.   In a mixing bowl, whisk together almond flour, cayenne pepper, pepper, mustard, salt, and xanthan gum.

4.   Slowly add heavy cream and mix until well combined.

5.   Whisk in fresh egg yolks, chives, and cheese until well combined.

6.   In a bowl, add fresh egg whites and cream of tartar and beat until stiff peaks form.

7.   Gently fold fresh egg white mixture into the almond flour mixture until well combined.

8.   Pour mixture into the prepared ramekins and place on cookie sheet.

9.   Bake in preheated oven for 210 minutes or until lightly golden brown.

10.   Serve hot and enjoy.

Lentil Curry Soup

INGREDIENT

- 2 teaspoon of kosher salt
- 1/2 teaspoon turmeric powder
- 1/9 to 1/2 teaspoon of cayenne pepper is used more for seasoning or is dropped if the seasoning is sensitive
- 2 jar of coconut milk (2 4 oz)
- 2 teaspoons of fresh lemon fresh Juice squeeze about 1 lemon
- Brown rice prepared for serving
- One and half cups brown or green lentils
- 1 tablespoon coconut oil
- 2 cup plus 2 teaspoon of chia water
- 2 chopped purple bulb
- 4 st. Spoons of chopped fresh ginger
- 2 teaspoons chopped garlic about 6 fresh cloves

- one tablespoon curry powder
- Half teaspoon of coconut sugar. Brown sugar is an alternative

DIRECTIONS

1. Rinse and drain, then set aside. Put the instant utensils to fry and add the coconut oil.
2. After the butter melts, add 2 tablespoon of water, shallots, ginger and garli
3. Cook often and stir until fragrant and the onions are soft, about 5 minutes.
4. Add curry powder, coconut sugar, salt, turmeric and cayenne pepper and stir vigorously.
5. Stop and try not to inhale the vapors coming from the boiler (tear gas!).
6. Add lentils, coconut milk and 4 cup of water.
7. Stir well so that the liquid completely covers the lentils.

8. Press the cancel button to stop frying, cover with a lid, then set to cook at high pressure for 35 minutes.

9. (It will take about 8 minutes to press, after which the timer will start.) When the timer stops, allow the pressure to naturally decrease for 25 minutes, then release to relieve the full pressure full.

10. Get the lid opened, include lemon fresh Juice and mix properly.

11. Season and adjust spices as desired. If the curry is too thick, add a little more water to fluff as needed.

12. Serve hot with rice, sprinkled with coriander.

Tools For Making A Quick Pot Of Pumpkin Cream Soup

Ingredient

- One (fifteen ounce) jar of fresh tomato sauce
- 2 teaspoons honey or maple syrup (optional, skip 4 0)
- One liter of broth, chicken or vegetable
- 2 teaspoon garlic powder
- ¼ teaspoon of cinnamon
- 2 ½ teaspoon of kosher salt
- ¾ cups of creamy coconut milk (jars)
- 2 medium purple bulb, finely chopped
- 2 cups sweet potatoes peeled, chopped

- 2 jars (35 ounces) of pumpkin puree (not filled with pumpkin pie)

DIRECTION

1. Add onion, sweet potato, pumpkin, fresh tomato sauce, honey (if used), stewed chicken, garlic powder, cinnamon and salt in a 6-liter electric pressure cooker.
2. Close the lid tightly, select manual adjustment and set to high pressure for 8 minutes.
3. When the pressure cooker timer is set, quickly depressurize.
4. Add coconut milk. Using a dipped blender, grind until well combined and very smooth. If you do not have a shredder, carefully scoop the cooked fresh tomato mixture into a blender while kneading. Be sure to cover

tightly, cover with a towel and stir until well combined and very smooth.

5. Season and add salt if desired.

Instant Lentil Soup

Ingredient

- 1 teaspoon smoked chili powder
- 1 teaspoon chopped red pepper
- 2 jar (28 ounces) of diced tomatoes with their fresh Juice
- 2 cup brown or green lentils
- 4 cups vegetable broth
- 2 teaspoon salt
- 2 cups chopped spinach
- 1 cup chopped parsley
- 1 lemon, fresh Juice
- 1/2 cup olive oil
- 2 onion, chopped
- 4 carrots, chopped
- 4 sticks of celery, chopped
- 4 chopped garlic fresh cloves
- 2 teaspoons dill
- 2 teaspoon curry powder
- 1 teaspoon dried thyme

DIRECTION

1. Turn on the instant cookware and press the saute.
2. Add olive oil, onion, carrot and celery and cook for about 10 minutes until vegetables are tender.
3. Add garlic and spices, then click "cancel".
4. Add tomatoes with juice, lentils, broth and salt, and cover with a lid.
5. Cook the soup under high pressure for 35 minutes.
6. When finished, turn the vents and let the pressure drop naturally for 30 to 35 minutes.
7. Gently remove the skin, then put 2 cups of soup in a blender and puree until sour cream.
8. Add to the soup with chopped spinach and cover.

9. Leave for 5 to 10 minutes until the spinach is wilted.
10. Just before serving, mix the chopped lemon fresh Juice and parsley and serve!

Pumpkin Bean Soup

INGREDIENT

- 2 teaspoon of olive oil
- 2 chopped purple bulb
- 2 carrot, chopped
- 2 celery rib, chopped
- 4 fresh cloves chopped garlic
- 4 pounds of chopped peeled zucchini (about 2 medium size zucchini)
- 4 cups vegetable broth

- 2 green apple, peeled, seeds and chopped
- ¼ teaspoon of ground cinnamon
- 2 teaspoon of kosher salt
- ¼ teaspoon of black pepper
- A pinch of nutmeg, if desired
- 2 fresh thyme
- 2 fresh rosemary

DIRECTIONS

1. Choose a stir-fry on your instant pot.
2. Add the olive oil and simmer the onions, carrots, celery and garlic until cooked through, about 5 to 10 minutes.
3. Add vegetable broth, pumpkin, apple, nutmeg, cinnamon, thyme, rosemary, salt, pepper and nutmeg, if used.
4. Securely place the lid on the instant dish and slide the handle to cover tightly.

5. Cook under high pressure for 25 minutes and quickly release the pressure.
6. Use a dip in an instant pot blender to puree the soup until smooth.
7. If you do not have a blender, you can let the soup cool down a bit and carefully transfer the soup to a regular blender and grind until smooth.

Summer Fresh Tomato Soup

INGREDIENT

- 2 cup vegetable broth with low sodium content

72

- 2 tablespoon kosher salt
- Serving options: freshly ground black pepper, butter
- 4 pounds of ripe tomatoes (about 6 large)
- 2 medium fresh onion
- 1/2 cup fresh basil leaves, and more to serve

DIRECTION

1. Cut 4 pounds of ripe tomatoes in half around the equator.
2. On a bowl, place a sieve with a fine mesh.
3. Using your fingers, scoop the fresh tomato seeds into a sieve and remove the fresh Juice from the bottom (approximately 1 cup of juice).
4. Remove the fresh tomato seeds. Place the jar scraper in a bowl and plan to cut out half of the fresh tomato over the small holes in the extractor.

5. Skin removal. You should have about 4 glasses of fresh tomato pulp and juice.

6. Chop 5 medium purple fresh onion (about 1/2 cup) and add to the pulp.

7. Place the freezer bag on the freezer inside the Instant Pot or electric pressure cookers.

8. Include 1/2 cup fresh basil leaves, shallots and fresh tomato pulp, one cup low-sodium vegetable broth and one tablespoon kosher salt into the bag.

9. Seal the bag and expel as much air as possible.

10. Freeze (bag inside the insert) until solid, at least 6-6 ½ hours or overnight.

11. Remove the bag from the insert and keep frozen for up to 4 months.

12. To cook, remove the frozen ingredients from the package and place in an instant bowl.

13. Lock the cover and make sure the pressure valve is closed.

14. Put to boil under high pressure for 10 minutes.

15. It will take 25 to 30 minutes to create pressure. When the cooking time is over, quickly relieve the pressure.

16. Use forceps to remove basil leaves. Beat the soup to combine.

17. Serve with freshly chopped basil leaves, ground black pepper and a little cream if desired.

Steel Cut Oats

INGREDIENT

- 1 teaspoon monosodium glutamate. kosher salt
- 2 st. maple syrup, and more to serve
- 2 teaspoon. pure vanilla extract
- Slice the bananas for serving
- Blueberries, serve
- Sliced chopped almonds for serving
- 2 S. oats cut out of steel
- 4 1 Country
- 2 2% milk
- 1 teaspoon monosodium glutamate. ground cinnamon

DIRECTIONS

1. Combine oats, water, milk, cinnamon and salt in an instant bowl.
2. Tap the manual setting and set the high cooking time to 10 minutes.
3. Allow the steam to come out naturally for 25 minutes before turning on the drain valve.
4. Cover and add maple syrup and vanilla to mix.
5. Serve with maple syrup, banana, blueberries and almonds.

Creamy And Light Humus

INGREDIENT

BEANS:

- 25 glasses of filtered water
- 2 kg of dried garbanzo beans

HUMUS:

- 2 medium fresh cloves of garlic
- 2 lemon
- 2 teaspoon of kosher salt
- 1 teaspoon dill
- 1/2 teaspoon smoked chili powder
- 1/2 cup of the highest quality olive oil
- 4 cups of boiled garbanzo beans are still warm
- 1 cup warm bean water for cooking
- 1/2 cup tahini

78

DIRECTION

1. Rinse the garbanzo beans and remove the ice. Place in an instant pot pan with 25 glasses of water.
2. Close the lid, make sure the vent is set to "airtight", and put the instant dishes in manual mode for 50 minutes.
3. Let the Instant Pot naturally lower the pressure when it runs.
4. If you press for time, let the IP reduce the natural pressure for at least 35 minutes, and then perform a quick and slow depressurization.
5. Rinse the bean fresh Juice thoroughly, making sure to keep the liquid!

Humus:

1. Transfer 4 cups of warm, dried garbanzo beans to a blender bowl with the blade attached.
2. Add all ingredients except olive oil.
3. Process until smooth and slowly add the olives through a test tube, once each time.
4. Hummus should be smooth, creamy and almost whipped to taste.
5. Serve with Za'atar, smoked chili powder and a little olive oil and enjoy!

Black Beans And Fresh Avocado

INGREDIENT

- 2 teaspoon cumin seeds
- 2 teaspoon cumin seeds
- 1 - 2 teaspoon chili powder
- 2 teaspoon of dry lime powder
- 2 teaspoon coriander
- 1 teaspoon turmeric
- 2 st. Spoon fresh tomato puree
- 2 can of chopped tomatoes (about 2 4 ounces)
- 2 block of vegetables
- 2-3 tablespoons of charisma to taste
- Season with fresh parsley or cilantro
- 250 g of dried chickpeas soaked in plenty of cold water for at least 4 hours (1 cup)
- Peel 4 -4 medium-sized carrots and cut into 2 -inch pieces

- 5 to 10 wax potatoes, peel and cut into 2 .6 inch pieces
- Oil spray
- 2 onion, chopped

DIRECTION

1. Heat your instant pot in saute mode and spray vigorously.
2. Add the onions and cook for 1 to 5 minutes until soft, stirring often and then seasoning.
3. Mix well, then add the ground tomatoes and canned tomatoes.
4. Add 1 jar of water from an empty jar of tomatoes.
5. Moisten pre-soaked chickpeas and place in a saucepan with carrots and potatoes.
6. Mint the broth in water and stir well and dip the vegetables in the liquid.

7. Close the lid, close the valve, cancel the Sauté mode, then cook in High manual mode for 25 minutes, and when the alarm sounds.
8. Stir well, season with spices, and then let Harrissa eat. Sprinkle with optional herbs and serve.

Black Garlic Beans

INGREDIENTS

- 2 sprig of esopate (Mexican grass), if any
- 2-3 fresh cloves of garlic
- 1 teaspoon dill seeds
- Salt after cooking
- Black beans 2 hand, soak overnight or soak quickly
- 1/2 cup water
- 2 piece of seaweed combo is 4 to 6 inches long

DIRECTIONS

1. Add the soaked beans, water, combo, garlic, herbs and spices to the pressure cooker.
2. Provides high pressure at strong heating.

3. Begin timing when the button lights up,.

4. After 10 minutes, remove the pot from the heat and let the pressure drop naturally.

5. Taste the beans to make sure the beans are done.

6. If not, put them back on the fire and reduce the pressure for a minute or two.

7. Repeat, bringing them to pressure and letting the pressure fall naturally.

8. Open the pot, tilt the lid away from you. Remove the combo and epazot. Salted beans to taste.

Mashed Potatoes

Ingredient

- 1 (2 stick) butter, add more to serve
- 1 Milk
- 1 sour cream
- Freshly ground black pepper
- 4 pounds Russian potatoes, peeled and forked
- 2 Country
- Salt beehive

Directions

1. Immediately place the potatoes, water and a pinch of salt in the pot.
2. Place the lid on the instant cookware and set the manual adjustment time, high, and set to 25 minutes.
3. When finished, turn on the quick discharge valve.

4. Drain the remaining liquid and transfer the potatoes to a bowl.

5. Use a mashed potato mill to a puree state.

6. Meanwhile, melt the butter and milk in a small saucepan over medium heat until heated.

7. Pour mashed potatoes and stir well to sour cream.

8. Mix in sour cream and use salt and pepper to season.

9. Transfer the potatoes to a serving bowl and cover with butter. Season with pepper.

Portobello Roast

INGREDIENT

- 4 cups of vegetable broth, separated
- Half cup white wine or dry red
- 4 teaspoons fresh tomato powder
- 2 tablespoons Worcestershire vegetarian sauce *
- 2 tablespoons cornstarch
- Freshly beat black pepper and Kosher salt
- Decorative options: chopped fresh parsley
- 2 .26 pounds of yellow Yukon potatoes, sliced to taste
- 2 pound of bell mushrooms (cut in half if large)
- 2 carrots, peel and cut into slices to taste
- 2 cups frozen fresh onion pearls *

- Four fresh cloves of garliThey should peeled and chopped
- 4 branches of fresh thyme

DIRECTION

1. Put potatoes, mushrooms, carrots, onions, garlic, thyme, 2.6 cups of vegetable broth, wine, fresh tomato sauce and pomegranate seeds in a ceramic bowl, then gently shake. Cook over low heat for 6-8 hours or over high heat for 4 -4 hours until potatoes and carrots are tender.
2. In a separate bowl, mix 1 cup of remaining vegetables and cornstarch until combined.
3. Add to the baking mixture and gently shake to combine.
4. Continue cooking for 5-10 minutes until the sauce thickens slightly.
5. Serve quickly, use fresh parsley to garnish if desired.

Measurement Method:

1. Place potatoes, mushrooms, carrots, onions, garlic, thyme, 2.6 cups of vegetable broth, wine, ketchup and pomegranate seeds in a pressure cooker bowl and mix gently. evenly.
2. Close the lid tightly and set the vent to "Sealed".
3. Press "Manual", then press "Pressure" until the "High Pressure" indicator lights up, and then adjust the up / down arrow until the reading time is 25 minutes.
4. Cooking. Then allow the pressure to discharge naturally, for about 35 minutes.
5. Carefully turn the vent to the "Ventilation" position, only to relieve any pressure that may still be inside. Remove the cover.

6. In a separate bowl, mix 1 cup of remaining vegetables and cornstarch until combined.
7. Add to the baking mixture and gently shake to combine.
8. Continue cooking for 2 -4 minutes until the sauce thickens slightly.
9. Serve quickly; use fresh parsley to garnish if desired.

Porridge

Ingredients

6 black peppercorns

salt

2 fresh cloves

45 g fine oat flakes

2 teaspoons of cinnamon powder

2 liter of milk

2 teaspoon ground turmeric

4 dates

8 tbsp heavy cream

2 teaspoons whole aniseed

4 tbsp blueberry spread

6 capsules of cardamom

2 tbsp coconut oil

Preparation:

1. Mortar the pepper, anise, fresh cloves
    and cardamom.

2. Then mix in the cinnamon and turmeriRoast the spices in a saucepan.

3. Deglaze the whole thing with 250 ml of water, bring to the boil and simmer for 10 minutes.

4. In the meantime, core the dates and roughly chop them.

5. Pour the water with the spices through a fine sieve.

6. Mix the water with the milk and bring to the boil.

7. Then stir in the dates and oatmeal. Let everything boil down for 25 minutes over medium heat. Stirring occasionally.

8. Finally season with salt and stir in the coconut oil.

9. To serve, spread the blueberry spread and 2 tablespoons of cream on each.

Homemade Granola

Ingredients

2 tsp spirulina powder

45 g coconut oil

salt

65 g quinoa

250 ml maple syrup

65 g flaked almonds

2 teaspoon ground cinnamon

65 g cashew nuts

45 g dried aronia berries

45 g coconut chips

250 g of oatmeal

Preparation:

1. Preheat the oven to 255 ° C fan oven.
2. Liquefy the coconut oil.
3. Rinse the quinoa with hot water through a sieve and dry.
4. Mix all ingredients except the spirulina powder and the quinoa.
5. Then spread on a baking sheet lined with baking paper.
6. Pour the quinoa on top and bake in the oven for 4 6 –45 minutes.
7. Stir every 25 minutes.
8. Finally let everything cool down and fold in the spirulina powder.

Buttermilk Pancakes

Ingredients

4 teaspoons of tartar baking powder
2 fresh eggs
2 pinch of salt
65 g of liquid butter
2 tbsp oil
250 g chopped walnuts
25 tbsp maple syrup
265 g wheat flour
4 8 6 ml buttermilk

Preparation:

1. Mix together baking powder, flour, salt and 65 g walnuts.
2. Mix the buttermilk, butter, fresh eggs and 2 tbsp maple syrup together.
3. Then fold in the nut-flour mixture and let it soak for 25 minutes.

4. Put the oil in a pan and bake the dough in portions on both sides.
5. Serve the finished pancakes with the maple syrup and walnuts.

Breakfast Jam

Ingredients

250 ml apple fresh Juice
2 kg of apples
250 ml apple cider
280 g fresh ginger
650 g preserving sugar
Fresh Juice of 2 lemons

Preparation:

1. Peel, core and dice the apples.
2. Peel and also dice the ginger. Put everything together in a saucepan and bring to the boil.
3. Let simmer for 10 minutes.
4. Stir again and again.
5. Then take the pot off the stove and pour the jam into containers that have been rinsed with hot water.
6. After sealing, turn the container upside down for 10 minutes.

Sunflower Sprout Muesli

Ingredients

480 g yogurt
4 tbsp almond sticks
6 tbsp buckwheat grains
4 teaspoons of raisins
8 tbsp sunflower sprouts
255 ml sweet cream
2 red apples
2 tbsp honey
4 oranges
2 teaspoon ground bourbon vanilla
2 bananas

Preparation:

1. Let the buckwheat grains soak overnight.

2. Then rinse them cold with the sunflower sprouts.
3. Cut the fruit into small pieces.
4. Mix the vanilla with the yogurt and honey.
5. Whip the cream until stiff and fold in the buckwheat, raisins and almond sticks.
6. Put the yoghurt mixture in a bowl to serve. Put the fruits and sprouts on top.

Bread Rolls For Breakfast

Ingredients

450 ml of lukewarm water
2 teaspoon honey

2 yeast cube

65 g margarine

465 g wheat meal

2-3 teaspoons of sea salt

Preparation:

1. Mix the yeast and honey with a little water.
2. Put the meal in a bowl and make a well in the middle.
3. Put the yeast mixture in this and mix in some grist.
4. Let it rise for 35 minutes.
5. Mix the margarine with the remaining water and salt and add.
6. Let it rise for 45 minutes.
7. Knead the dough and shape it into rolls.
8. Let this rise again for 50 minutes.
9. Then scratch lightly and sprinkle with the seeds if desired.

10. Bake the rolls for 45 minutes at 250°

Buttermilk drink

Ingredients

250 g fresh wheat meal

8 65 ml buttermilk

4 tbsp flaxseed

4 tbsp unsweetened sea buckthorn

2 tbsp honey

Preparation:

1. Mix the honey with the buttermilk and the sea buckthorn.
2. Stir in the flaxseed and the crushed wheat and season to taste.

Hearty Breakfast

Ingredients

2 tbsp butter

65 g mushrooms

2 fresh onion

1 red pepper

4 fresh eggs

4 jacket potatoes

1 bunch of chives

Preparation:

1. Peel the jacket potatoes, cut into slices and fry in the butter.
2. Chop the onions and add them to the potatoes.
3. Season the whole thing with salt and pepper.
4. Clean the mushrooms and peppers and cut into strips.
5. Whisk the fresh eggs .

6. Raise everything to the potatoes and stir.
7. Let the whole thing stand for about 10 minutes.

Cherry Pudding With Cereal Porridge

Ingredients

1 glass of sweet cherries
250 ml of sweet cream
2 tbsp vanilla pudding powder
2 tbsp almond flakes
250 g natural yogurt
80 g of ground wheat
2 tbsp bourbon vanilla sugar

Preparation:

1. Let the crushed wheat swell overnight.
2. Then pour off the water.
3. Catch approx. 280 ml of cherry fresh Juice from the cherries.
4. Heat the fresh Juice and stir in the pudding.
5. Let everything cool and fold in the cherries.
6. Toast the almond flakes in a pan.
7. Beat the cream with the sugar until stiff.
8. Mix half of the cream with the wheat.
9. Mix the rest of the cream with the yogurt.
10. Layer everything alternately in bowls and sprinkle with the flaked almonds.

Fruit Pulp

Ingredients

- 2 25 g of grapes
- 450 g yogurt
- 6 tbsp breakfast porridge
- 450 ml orange-mango syrup
- 65 g walnuts
- 2 pears
- 2 teaspoon cinnamon

Preparation:

1. Cut the pears into cubes.
2. Mix the pulp with the fresh Juice and bring to the boil.
3. Then mix in the cinnamon and yogurt.
4. Arrange the porridge.
5. Spread the fruits and walnuts on top.

Blueberry Mint Muesli

Ingredients

2 teaspoon acai powder
255 g whole grain muesli
2 tbsp sliced almonds
2 stalk of mint
65 g blueberries
2 teaspoon honey
250 g yogurt

Preparation:

1. Wash, dry and freeze the berries.
2. Mix the yogurt with the honey and the acai powder.
3. Divide the muesli together with the almonds in bowls and pour the yoghurt mixture on top.
4. Finally, arrange the frozen berries with the mint on top.

Buckwheat Porridge With Fruits

Ingredients

250 g raspberries

250 g blueberries

2 pinch of cinnamon

65 grams of sugar

For the porridge:

250 g of sugar

2 fresh egg white

250 ml of water

2 teaspoon butter

250 g buckwheat

Preparation:

1. Heat the buckwheat and fresh egg white in a saucepan.
2. Stir constantly.

3. Drain the water when the fresh egg white has set.
4. Then stir in the sugar and simmer for 35 minutes.
5. Stir the butter into the finished pulp.
6. Caramelize the sugar for the fruit with 2 tablespoons of water.
7. Add 2 tbsp water and the fruit and heat briefly.
8. Finally add the cinnamon and serve together.

Fresh Egg And Cucumber Spread

Ingredients

salt and pepper
2 tbsp rapeseed oil
280 g cucumber
25 g low-fat quark

2 bunch of fresh herbs

4 slices of wholemeal bread
2 tsp hot mustard
2 fresh eggs

Preparation:

1. Hard-boil the fresh eggs , rinse and cool. Halve the cucumber lengthways, remove the seeds and cut into small pieces together with the herbs.
2. Peel the fresh eggs .
3. Dice the fresh egg white, mash the fresh egg yolk.
4. Mix the quark with the fresh egg yolk, mustard and oil.
5. Fold the cucumber with the fresh egg white and herbs into the quark.
6. Season everything with salt and pepper.

Fruit Spice Bread

Ingredients

2 tsp germ oil
2 small stick of leek
2 apple
2 slices of wholemeal spelled bread
450 g flour boiling potatoes
salt and pepper
4 marjoram stalks

Preparation:

1. Wash the potatoes and cook with the skin on for 20–45 minutes.
2. Wash the marjoram and pluck the leaves.
3. Chop the leaves, except for a few.
4. Halve the leek lengthways, wash and cut into strips.
5. Wash and dice the apple.

6. Heat the oil in a pan and steam the leek for about 10 minutes.

7. Add the apple and the chopped marjoram and cook for 2 minute.

8. Season everything with salt and pepper.

9. Rinse, peel and press the finished potatoes.

10. Then fold in the apple mixture.

11. Season everything with salt and pepper.

12. Put the spread on the bread slices and serve with the remaining marjoram.

Classic Rice Pudding

Ingredients

250 g short grain rice
2 handful of raisins
2 tbsp vanilla sugar
2 tbsp brown sugar
650 ml of milk
2 teaspoon cinnamon

Preparation:

1. Bring the milk to the boil, along with the rice, vanilla sugar, raisins and rice.
2. Reduce the heat and cook for about 65 minutes.
3. Stir occasionally.
4. Fill the finished rice pudding into bowls and sprinkle with cinnamon and sugar before serving.

A little different breakfast fresh eggs

Ingredients

- 4 fresh eggs
- 2 pinch of salt

Preparation:

1. Boil the fresh eggs for 5 minutes.
2. Then take it out and open it. Put the yolks in an extra glass.
3. Remove the fresh egg white and add to the fresh egg yolk.
4. Mix everything gently and season with salt.

Omelette With Goat Cheese

Ingredients

- 2 tbsp basil
- salt and pepper
- 250 g goat cheese
- 65 g butter
- 4 fresh eggs

Preparation:

1. Beat the fresh eggs .
2. Season with salt and pepper and whisk.
3. Dice the goat cheese.
4. Chop the basil.
5. Add both to the fresh eggs . Heat half of the butter in a pan.
6. Put half of the fresh egg mixture in the pan and let it set.

7. Then fold the omelette in the middle and serve. Do the same for the second omelette.

Raw Vegetables With Fruits

Ingredients

1 mango
salt and pepper
1 apple
65 g yogurt
Lemon fresh Juice
2 tbsp pumpkin seeds
250 g celery root
2 tbsp honey

Preparation:

1. Peel the celery. Cut into strips with the apple.
2. Drizzle both with lemon juice.
3. Mix the yogurt with salt and pepper.
4. Add the yogurt to the apple. Peel and core the mango and cut into wedges.
5. Marinate the mango in lemon fresh Juice and honey.
6. Roast the pumpkin seeds in a pan without fat.
7. Arrange the celery and mango.
8. Scatter the pumpkin seeds on top.

Fruity Spread

Ingredients

80 g cereal
2 tbsp lemon fresh Juice
80 g cream cheese
65 g honey

2 banana

250 g yogurt

2 tbsp fresh orange fresh Juice

Preparation:

1. Mix the yogurt with the honey and both types of juice.
2. Then fold in the muesli and let it steep for 2 hours.
3. Mash the banana and fold into the yoghurt along with the cream cheese.

Baked Toast

Ingredients

salt and pepper

2 tbsp olive oil

2 clove of garlic

2 tbsp basil pesto

4 slices of toast

2-3 tomatoes

Fresh basil

2 pk. Mozzarella

Preparation:

1. Wash the tomatoes and cut into slices along with the mozzarella.
2. Chop the garliBrush the toast with pesto.
3. Place the tomatoes and mozzarella on top.
4. Mix the olive oil with the garlic and pour over it.
5. Baked the toasts in the oven.
6. Garnish the finished toasts with the basil.

Pomegranate Granola

Ingredients

4 tbsp wheat germ
2 tbsp lemon fresh Juice
2 pomegranate
2 tbsp raisins
265 ml buttermilk
2 oranges
25 tbsp wholegrain oat flakes
2 kiwis
2 tbsp honey

Preparation:

1. Fillet the oranges. Peel and cut the kiwi fruit.
2. Add the raisins and lemon juice.

3. Mix the honey and buttermilk together.
4. Add the oat flakes and wheat germ to the fruit.
5. Then add the buttermilk.
6. Core the pomegranate.
7. Put the seeds under the muesli.

Vegetable Muesli

Ingredients

2 apple
6 tbsp fine oat flakes
Lemon fresh Juice
265 g low-fat natural yogurt
2 tbsp honey
2 carrot
2 tbsp chopped walnuts

Preparation:

1. Grate the carrot and apple.
2. Drizzle both with a little lemon juice.
3. Mix the yogurt with the oatmeal.
4. Then add the carrot and apple.
5. Season everything with honey.

Fresh Egg In A Pepper Ring

Ingredients

2 bell pepper
salt and pepper
2 fresh eggs
chopped herbs

Preparation:

1. Wash and core the peppers and cut into two rings.
2. Heat oil in a pan.
3. Put the peppers inside.
4. Beat an fresh egg into each of the pepper rings.
5. Let the fresh egg freeze.
6. Then carefully remove and serve.

Waffles With Coconut

Ingredients

250 g corn starch
250 g butter
250 g desiccated coconut
250 g of sugar
250 ml of water
250 g flour
4 fresh eggs

Preparation:

1. Mix all of the above ingredients into a dough. Bake the waffles in portions in a waffle iron.

Overnight Oatmeal Porridge

Ingredients

4 tbsp oatmeal
2 handful of raisins
2 tbsp chia seeds
250 ml of milk
2 tbsp desiccated coconut

Preparation:

1. Warm up the milk.
2. Add the oatmeal and bring to the boil.
3. Then add the chia seeds, raisins and desiccated coconut.
4. Mix everything together and let it soak overnight.
5. The next day, cut the fruit into small pieces and add to the pulp.

Breakfast Fruit Fresh Juice

Ingredients

2 lime
4 handfuls of spinach leaves
2 avocados

265 g coconut milk
2 pineapple

Preparation:

1. Peel and cut the pineapple.
2. Wash the spinach.
3. Peel and halve the lime and avocados.
4. Fresh Juice these ingredients and mix with the coconut milk.

Toasted Bread With Pear

Ingredients

4 pears
250 g Greek yogurt
2 tbsp chopped hazelnuts
Lemon balm
4–8 slices of spelled bread
4 tbsp maple syrup

Preparation:

1. Mix the yogurt with 2 tablespoons of maple syrup.
2. Peel the pear and cut into wedges.
3. Toast the bread.
4. Spread the yoghurt on the bread and spread the pears on top.
5. Finally, sprinkle with lemon balm and hazelnuts.

131

Papaya Smoothie

Ingredients

2 tbsp chia seeds

Fresh Juice of 2 grapefruits

2–4 tbsp coconut flakes

Fresh Juice of a lime

250 ml buttermilk

250 ml coconut milk

2 dash of maple syrup

2 mango

2 tbsp cornflowers

2 papaya

Preparation:

1. Peel and cut the fruit.
2. Puree all ingredients.
3. Fill the smoothie into glasses to serve.

Rolled toast

Ingredients

4 pk. vanilla sugar

2 tbsp sugar

265 g quark (45 %)

25 slices of toast

65 g butter

2 fresh orange

2 fresh eggs

5 to 10 passion fruit

450 ml of milk

Preparation:

1. Mix the fresh eggs with the sugar and milk.
2. Soak the toast in it, drain and fry in a pan with fat on both sides.

133

3. Mix the quark with the vanilla sugar.
4. Halve the passion fruit, remove the stone and collect the juice.
5. Fold the fresh Juice and the stones into the quark.
6. Peel the orange.
7. Chop half of it and also fold it into the quark. Spread some quark on the toast and chill for 2-2 ½ hour.
8. Then roll the toasts and serve.

Buttermilk Shake With Kiwi

Ingredients

2 cups of buttermilk

Fresh Juice and zest of 1 lemon

6–8 tbsp maple syrup

2 tbsp turmeric

1 bunch of lemon balm

8 golden kiwi fruit

1 tonka bean

Preparation:

1. Peel the kiwi. Puree all ingredients. Pour the shake into glasses to serve.

Vegetable Jam

Ingredients

650 g zucchini

2 teaspoon gelling agent

65 ml of water

450 g of sugar
650 g sour apples

Preparation:

1. Peel, core and grate the zucchini.
2. Peel the apples and cut them into cubes.
3. Put both in a saucepan and boil for 8–25 minutes with water over low heat, then add the sugar and cook again for 6 –25 minutes.
4. Finally add the gelling agent according to the package instructions.
5. Take the finished jam off the stove and pour it into a container.

Chia Yogurt With Cinnamon

Ingredients

1 teaspoon cinnamon

2 apple

2 tbsp chia seeds

1 teaspoon honey

265 g natural yogurt

Preparation:

1. Mix the yogurt with cinnamon, honey and chia seeds and place in the refrigerator for 45 minutes.
2. In the meantime, cut the apple into small pieces and then fold it into the yogurt.

Sweet pancakes with cheese

Ingredients

- 65 g of cottage cheese
- 2 dash of almond milk
- 2 banana
- 2 pinch of baking powder
- 65 g oatmeal
- 2 tbsp natural yogurt
- 2 fresh egg
- some coconut oil

Preparation:

1. Puree the banana, almond milk, oat flakes, baking powder, fresh egg and the cottage cheese together.
2. Heat some coconut oil in a pan and fry the pancakes in portions on both sides.

3. Spread the yogurt and fruit over the top before serving.

Toasted Bread With Avocado Strips

Ingredients

2 avocado
80 g of cottage cheese
2 teaspoon lemon fresh Juice
2 slices of dark bread
salt and pepper

Preparation:

1. Toast the bread first. Peel the avocado and cut into strips.
2. Spread the cottage cheese on the toasted bread and top with the avocado strips.

3. Finally, season with the lemon juice, salt and pepper.

Sweet Potatoes

Ingredients

1 bunch of parsley
4 fresh eggs
salt and pepper
Chilli flakes
2 sweet potatoes
250 g of grainy cream cheese
2 spring onions

Preparation:

1. Wash the sweet potatoes and cut in half lengthways.

2. Place the potato halves on a baking sheet and bake for 4 0–45 minutes at 250 ° In the meantime, wash the spring onions and cut into rings.
3. Hollow out the finished sweet potatoes a little.
4. Open an fresh egg in this recess and season with salt and pepper.
5. Scatter the spring onions on top. Bake the whole thing again for 35 minutes.
6. Wash and chop the parsley.
7. Serve everything with a little cream cheese and sprinkle with the parsley and chilli flakes before serving.

Fast Sandwiches

Ingredients

2 spring onions
1 cucumber
4 tbsp mayonnaise
2 lemon
4 tbsp yogurt
2 bunch of rocket
2 fresh eggs
8 slices of toast

Preparation:

1. Boil the fresh eggs for 8 minutes.
2. Then quench, peel and cut into small pieces.
3. Chop the spring onions and mix together with the zest and fresh Juice of the lemon, fresh eggs , mayonnaise and yoghurt.

144

4. Taste everything. Peel and slice the cucumber.
5. Salt these and let them steep for 25 minutes.
6. Brush the toast slices with the mayonnaise mixture.
7. Squeeze out the cucumber and divide with the rocket on 4 slices of toast.
8. Then place the other slices on top.

Smoothie To Spoon

Ingredients

2 tbsp chia seeds
280 g mixed berries
250 ml of milk
2 dates
2 tbsp coconut chips
2 banana

2 tbsp almonds
250 g mango

Preparation:

1. Peel the banana and mango.
2. Put some of the fruit aside.
3. Puree the rest with the milk and dates.
4. Then add the chia seeds and let soak for 35 minutes.
5. Finally put everything in a bowl.
6. Spread the fruit, almonds and coconut chips on top.

Fried White Beans

Ingredients

2 fresh onion
2 tbsp coarse mustard
2 clove of garlic
2 tbsp balsamic vinegar
2 tablespoons oil
2 tbsp sugar beet syrup
265 ml vegetable broth
2 clove
2 bay leaf
5-10 fresh eggs
450 g dried white beans
Cayenne pepper
850 g peeled tomatoes
salt

Preparation:

1. Soak the beans in cold water overnight.
2. The next day, cover the beans in a saucepan with water, bring to the boil and simmer for 45 minutes.
3. In the meantime, dice the tomatoes and onions.
4. Chop the garliThen drain the beans.
5. Heat oil in a pan.
6. Stew the garlic and onions in it.
7. Add all ingredients except the fresh eggs .
8. Bring the whole thing to the boil and simmer for 45 minutes.
9. Season with salt and pepper, remove the clove and bay leaf.
10. Fry the fresh eggs in a separate pan with oil.

Omelette With Herbs

Ingredients

salt and pepper

25 tbsp herbs

1/9 L milk

6 tbsp butter

2 tbsp parmesan

25 fresh eggs

2 tbsp flour

Preparation:

1. Melt the butter in a pan. Steam the herbs in it.
2. Mix the fresh eggs with the parmesan, milk, flour, salt and pepper.
3. Pour the dough over the herbs and stir. Bake the omelette on both sides.

Filled Flatbread

Ingredients

2 avocados
250 ml vegetable stock
ground cumin
salt and pepper
2 tbsp lemon fresh Juice
sugar
2 tbsp fresh orange fresh Juice
4 smooth parsley stalks
2 clove of garlic
2 flat breads
2 red peppers
4 mint stalks
2 fresh onion
250 g yogurt
2 tbsp olive oil

Preparation:

1. Peel and core the peppers and cut into strips.
2. Peel the fresh onion and cut into strips.
3. Heat olive oil. Braise the fresh onion in it.
4. Then add the peppers. Deglaze with the stock.
5. Let everything simmer until the liquid has evaporated.
6. Then season with the spices. Wash and chop the parsley.
7. Add this to the pepper. Let everything cool down.
8. Peel the garlic, chop it finely and mix it with the lemon and fresh orange juice.
9. Season to taste with salt, pepper and cumin.
10. Peel the avocado and dice the pulp.

11.   Add the avocado to the fresh orange marinade and let it rest for 45 minutes.
12.   Mix the yogurt with salt and pepper.
13.   Chop the mint and add.
14.   Briefly heat the bread in the oven, cut in half and cut into it.
15.   Finally fill the bread.

Baked Fresh Eggs With Bread

Ingredients

2 red fresh onion
salt and pepper
2 tbsp oil
2 tbsp fresh tomato paste

2 tomatoes

2 pk. Feta

2 bell pepper

4 fresh eggs

2 bell pepper

oregano

Preparation:

1. Wash the peppers and tomatoes.
2. Dice both with the onion.
3. Heat oil in a pan.
4. Steam the onions in it. Then add the peppers.
5. Finally, stir in the tomatoes with the fresh tomato paste.
6. Season everything with salt, pepper and oregano and stir. Then put in a bowl.
7. Beat the fresh eggs in the same pan and fry them with fried fresh eggs.
8. Then pour the vegetables over it. Halve the feta.

9. Roughly distribute one half over the vegetables and the other half finely.
10. Close the pan and let the feta melt. Sprinkle with oregano before serving and serve with the bread.

Almond And Avocado Canapes

Ingredients

2 clove of garlic
2 lemon
2 sprig of thyme
250 g spring onions
4 tbsp donated almonds
450 g avocado
2 teaspoon honey
2 ciabatta bread
salt and pepper
2 teaspoons of olive oil

65 g radishes

Preparation:

1. Preheat the oven to 280° C fan oven.
2. Roast the almond sticks in the oven for 10 minutes.
3. Cut the bread into slices. Mix the garlic with the oil and drizzle the bread slices with it.
4. Then salt and sprinkle with thyme leaves.
5. Roast the ciabatta bread in the oven for 2 0–35 minutes. In the meantime, dice the avocado.
6. Wash the spring onions and cut into rings.
7. Put both in a bowl. Wash, squeeze and grate the lemon.
8. Add the lemon fresh Juice and the zest with the honey to the avocado.
9. Mix everything and season with salt and pepper.

10. Fold in the almonds and put everything together on the bread slices.
11. Wash and slice the radishes and pour them over the slices of bread.

Vegetable Butter

Ingredients

- 1 bunch of parsley
- 6 carrots
- salt
- 250 g cold butter

Preparation:

1. Peel, wash and dice the carrots.
2. Steam these in salted water and drain.
3. Wash the parsley leaves.

4. Puree all ingredients and season with salt.
5. Chill the butter before serving.

Mixed Bread

Ingredients

- 450 g of rye flour
- ½ tbsp sugar
- 250 g wheat meal
- 2 pk. Dry germ
- 850 ml of lukewarm water
- 450 g of wheat flour
- ½ tbsp salt

Preparation:

1. Mix all of the flour with the dried yeast and sugar. D
2. issolve the salt in the water.
3. Add the salted water to the flour and knead until it no longer sticks.

4. Then put the dough in a Roman pot and let it rise for 2 .6 hours in a warm place.
5. Then put the pot in the oven and bake for 2 hour at 250 °

Potato Rolls With Sugar

Ingredients

1/9 l skimmed milk
265 g floury potatoes
80 g low-fat yogurt
265 g wheat flour
2 fresh egg
265 g whole wheat flour
80 g of sugar
2 pack of dry yeast

Preparation:

1. Steam the potatoes with their skin on for 25 minutes.
2. Then peel and press.
3. Then add the sugar, yeast, flour, fresh egg and yoghurt.
4. Approx. Add 250 ml milk. Knead everything and let rise for 4 0-410 minutes in a warm place.
5. Then form rolls out of it and let rise for 25 minutes.
6. Finally, steam the rolls for 3 horas

Mexican Chilli Tortilla

Ingredients

6 fresh eggs
2 red chilli pepper
2 red pepper
250 g boiled kidney beans
2 25 g cooked sweet corn

olive oil

450 g waxy potatoes

salt and pepper

Preparation:

1. Peel the potatoes and cut into slices.
2. Fry these in oil and set aside.
3. Dice the peppers and fry them in the same way.
4. Whisk the fresh eggs . Add the potatoes, beans, corn and peppers.
5. Core and chop the chilli pepper.
6. Season the potato mixture with the chilli, salt and pepper.
7. In a pan, fry half of the mixture in oil on both sides. Cut the finished tortilla into quarters and serve.

Fresh Tomato Mozzarella Ciabatta

Ingredients

1/2 kg of diced tomatoes
2 loaf of ciabatta
2 fresh cloves of garlic
some olive oil
salt and pepper
2 handful of chopped basil
2 pinch of paprika powder
2-3 pk. Mozzarella

Preparation:

1. Fry the tomatoes and garlic in olive oil. Season everything with salt, sugar, paprika powder, basil and pepper.
2. Let everything stand for 10 minutes.
3. Put the whole thing on the ciabatta.

4. Cut the mozzarella into small pieces and spread on top.
5. Sprinkle with basil before serving.

Savory Muffins With Onions

Ingredients
butter
2 fresh onion
salt
250 g spelled flour
250 g of grated cheese
80 ml of vegetable oil
250 g buttermilk
1 teaspoon baking soda
2 teaspoons of baking soda
2 fresh egg

Preparation:

1. Grease the muffin pan.
2. Preheat the oven to 250 ° Peel and dice the onion.
3. Whisk the egg. Add oil and buttermilk.
4. Add the fresh onion and 1/2 of the cheese.
5. Then stir in the flour, baking soda and baking powder.
6. Pour 1/2 of the batter into the muffin tins.
7. Sprinkle the rest of the cheese on top.
8. Bake the muffins for 2 6 –25 minutes.
9. Let the muffins cool for 25 minutes before serving.

Curry Cream Cheese

Ingredients

6 dried apricots
250 g of grainy cream cheese
curry
2 spring onions
salt and pepper

Preparation:

1. Wash the spring onions and cut into rings. Dice the apricots.
2. Mix both with the cream cheese and season with salt, pepper and curry.

Amaranth And Quinoa Mixed Bread

Ingredients

450 ml of milk

250 g rye flour

1 teaspoon sugar

2 cube of yeast

2 1 teaspoons of salt

1 teaspoon caraway seeds

250 g quinoa

2 teaspoon ground coriander

65 g amaranth

450 g spelled flour

Preparation:

1. Toast the quinoa and amaranth in a pan.
2. Then add 250 ml milk and 450 ml water as well as the salt.

3.
4. Let everything cook for about 210 minutes.
5. Heat the rest of the oat milk with sugar.
6. Mix the yeast in it.
7. Drain the amaranth-quinoa mixture and add to the yeast together with both types of flour and the spices.
8. Knead everything and let rise for about 45 minutes in a warm place.
9. Grease a loaf pan and add the batter.
10. Let it rise for another 3 horas
11. Then bake for about 45 minutes at 250 ° C fan oven.

Blueberry Quinoa

Ingredients

8 65 ml unsweetened almond milk
2 cup blueberries (alternatively raspberries or strawberries)
2 handful of sunflower seeds
Apple syrup
2 handful of walnuts
1 teaspoon vanilla extract
65 g raisins
2 cup of quinoa
2 teaspoon cinnamon powder
2 small apple, cut into cubes

Preparation:

1. First, the quinoa is put in a saucepan with the almond milk and cinnamon.
2. After that, everything is brought to a boil.

3. As soon as the contents boil, the pot is covered.

4. Now the stove is put on a low flame so that the contents simmer gently.

5. Stir everything well from time to time so that nothing burns.

6. After everything has simmered again for 10 minutes, the apple cubes and the raisins are added.

7. Then everything has to simmer again for 10 minutes.

8. After the 10 minutes have elapsed, the pot is removed from the stove so that the contents can be drawn with the lid closed.

9. Now everything is seasoned with the apple syrup and the berries and nuts are stirred in.

10.   Then the blueberry quinoa can be served.

Muesli With Crunch

Ingredients

- 2 apples
- 2 tbsp agave syrup
- 4 teaspoons of tiger nuts
- 6 walnut halves
- 2 dates
- 2 ripe bananas
- Fresh Juice of half a lemon

Preparation:

1. First the bananas and apples are peeled.
2. The bananas are then cut into slices and the apples into small pieces.
3. The cut fruit is set aside in a bowl.
4. The dates are also cut into small pieces and the walnut halves roughly chopped.

5. Now the roughly chopped walnut halves are placed in a coated pan with the agave syrup and briefly roasted.
6. Then the walnut halves are mixed into the fruit together with the tiger nut flakes, lemon fresh Juice and dates.

The Fruity Bomb

Ingredients

2 kiwis
2 carrots
1 pineapple
2 pear

]Preparation:

1. The pineapple is peeled and cut into pieces.
2. The pieces should fit in a juicer later.
3. The carrots are brushed with a vegetable brush under running water and also cut into pieces for the juicer.
4. Likewise, the kiwi is peeled and cut into pieces for the juicer if necessary.
5. The pear is washed and pitted thoroughly.
6. Then it is cut into coarse cutlets.
7. Now the fruit fresh Juice is pressed through the juicer.
8. Fill this into a glass and enjoy the fruity bomb.

Porridge With Tiger Nuts

Ingredients

2 dried, unsulphurized figs
250 ml hot spring water
1 apple
2 banana
2 teaspoon of crushed flaxseed
4 tbsp organic tiger nut flakes

Preparation:

1. The tiger nut flakes are poured over with hot water, stirred and set aside to swell.
2. In the meantime, the banana can be peeled and mashed with a fork.
3. The apple is washed and finely grated.

4. The figs are also cut into small pieces.
5. Finally, the mashed bananas, the grated apple and the figs are added to the tiger nut flake porridge together with the flaxseed. For serving, the porridge is arranged in a bowl.

Porridge With Apple

Ingredients

2 tbsp oatmeal
cinnamon
2 tbsp almonds
milk
cardamom
4 tbsp buckwheat
2 apple

Preparation:

1. The almonds are roughly chopped and soaked in a little water with the buckwheat overnight and then rinsed through a sieve the next day.
2. The almonds and buckwheat are now put in a saucepan with the milk and oat flakes.
3. Everything is heated on a low flame with the pot closed.
4. In the meantime, the apple is grated and can be added to the porridge.
5. Finally, season everything with cardamom and cinnamon and serve warm.

Porridge With Coconut And Raspberries

Ingredients

480 ml milk
65 g desiccated coconut
2 tbsp rice syrup
salt
280 g raspberries
6 tbsp oatmeal
280 g red currants

Preparation:

1. First the good raspberries and currants are sorted out.
2. After that, they are washed, carefully patted dry and placed in a bowl.
3. Now the raspberries and currants are mixed together and set aside.

4. The milk is put in a saucepan with the oat flakes, desiccated coconut and a pinch of salt.
5. Bring everything to the boil briefly while stirring.
6. Then the porridge is removed from the stove to cool down.
7. For serving, the porridge is layered alternately with the berry mixture in a glass.
8. If you want, you can garnish everything with mint leaves.

Ginger And Cucumber Smoothie

Ingredients

- 2–4 tart apples
- 2 piece of ginger, finger length
- 2 handful of romaine lettuce
- 2 tbsp linseed oil
- 1 cucumber
- 2 handfuls of lamb's lettuce
- Water ad libitum

Preparation:

1. First the fruit, the cucumber and the lettuce leaves are washed.
2. The apples are then quartered and pitted.
3. The ginger is roughly chopped.

4. All ingredients are then placed in a tall vessel and pureed with a hand blender or stand mixer.

Omelette With Fresh Tomato

Ingredients

2 tbsp mineral water
2 dried tomatoes
4 fresh eggs
2 fresh tomatoes
2 tbsp rapeseed oil
2 shallot
salt and pepper

Preparation:

1. The shallot is peeled and diced. The dried tomatoes are cut into fine slices.
2. The fresh tomatoes are washed, halved and pitted.
3. Then they are cut into fine cubes.
4. Now the fresh eggs are whisked with salt, pepper and the mineral water.
5. Heat the oil in a pan and fry the shallots until golden.
6. Then add the fresh egg mixture and sprinkle with the tomatoes.
7. The fresh egg must now set on a mild heat.
8. Then the finished omelette can be halved and served on two plates.

Nettle Seed Soy Yogurt

Ingredients

2 tbsp nettle seeds

250 g yogurt

2 pinch of turmeric

2 tbsp flaxseed

2 tbsp linseed oil

2 tbsp wheat germ oil

8 6 g blueberries (fresh or frozen)

2 teaspoon rose hip powder

Preparation:

1. The blueberries are rinsed and patted dry.
2. Frozen blueberries must be thawed.
3. The yoghurt is stirred together with the oil.
4. The mixture can be made creamier with a little water if the oil is not enough as a liquid.

5. The turmeric, rose hip powder and nettle seeds are now mixed into the yoghurt.
6. The blueberries are poured over it for serving.

Banana And Nut Mash

Ingredients

- 45 ml of milk
- 2 banana
- 80 ml cashew milk
- 2 tbsp linseed oil
- 45 g tiger nut flakes

Preparation:

1. First mash the banana.
2. Then mix in the tiger nuts flakes.

3. Mix the whole thing with the milk and cashew milk. Finally stir in the linseed oil.

Apple And Nut Muesli

Ingredients

2 tbsp tiger nut flakes
4 almonds
2 walnuts
2 cup of yogurt / 2 apple
2 tbsp pumpkin seeds

Preparation:

1. Wash and dice the apple.
2. Chop the walnuts and almonds.
3. Mix both with the apple.
4. Roast the pumpkin seeds in a pan without fat and add them to the apple.

5. Then mix in the tiger nuts flakes.
6. Finally, stir everything together with the yogurt.

Fruit Bowl

Ingredients

2 banana
2 green apple
2 tbsp hemp flour
2 avocado

Preparation:

1. Halve the avocado and remove the stone.
2. Puree the pulp of the avocado with the banana.
3. Then add the hemp flour and stir. Dice the apple and add it.

4. Mix everything again.

Apricot Quinoa Mash

Ingredients:

450 ml of milk
6 apricots
2 tbsp pumpkin seeds
250 g quinoa

Preparation:

1. First wash and drain the quinoa.
2. Bring the milk to the boil and cook the quinoa in it for about 25 minutes.
3. In the meantime, halve the apricots and remove the stone.
4. Puree the apricot pulp.

5. Put the finished quinoa in a bowl and mix with the pureed apricots.

6. Finally, chop the pumpkin seeds and roast them in a pan without fat.

7. Sprinkle these over the apricot and quinoa mash.

CPSIA information can be obtained
at www.ICGtesting.com
Printed in the USA
BVHW041712190121
598137BV00012BB/879

9 781990 207211